RELEASING TRAUMA

From EMDR to M-REMB

Yoko Tanoue, M.D. , Ph.D.

Translated into English by Yoshikata Koga, Ph.D.

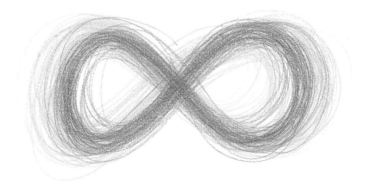

GENDAI SHOKAN

To my brother, Yoshikata Koga. Much thanks for your support.

Preface

I have served as a psychiatrist for the last fifty years, during the most recent thirty years of which I have operated a clinic which specializes in the care of children who require psychiatric treatment. In what follows, I will describe a treatment that actually worked, namely Eye Movement Desensitization and Reprocessing (EMDR). Now, I am sure this technique works well for children as well as adults.

However, there were cases where children have some difficulties following EMDR.

I feel it has limits. One problem is that EMDR reminds the patient of the reasons for PTSD, which can be painful. One more reason is that eye movements are necessary. Some toddlers cannot keep their eyes open. To cope with these difficulties, we removed the reminder about their traumatic experiences. In addition, to enhance the effects of eye movement, we applied Form Drawing, after Steiner's theory. (We show these results in Chapter III.) To ascertain the effect of our method, we added what we call " Image Breathing."

In short, "Image Breathing" is an exercise in which you imagine the situation in which you are the most comfortable. For example, you are lying on your back and watching clouds move, you are watching the vast sea, you are sitting on a bench in the woods, or you are watching stars and accepting the energy from the universe. For toddlers, an example might be that you are eating ice cream or your mom is holding you.

While you continue to imagine yourself in that state, start breathing out, shrinking your abdomen slowly at your own pace. Breath out slowly and empty your lungs completely. Depending on your situation, say (to yourself), "Breath out slowly until your lungs becomes empty." "Blow gently like you're softly blowing whistle," as if you want to elongate the blowing out time. For breathing in, relax your abdomen a little and the air will rush into your body.

This is our original method that we call M-REMB — Mental Release Eye Movement and Breathing.

RELEASING TRAUMA

From EMDR to M-REMB

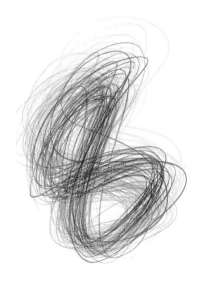

RELEASING TRAUMA

From EMDR to M-REMB

*

CONTENTS

CONTENTS

Chapter I

Form Drawing

Form Drawing; Enjoy Drawing

What to Prepare

Several pieces of white, A3-size paper and colored pencils or crayons. Use about five colors out of twelve. If you don't have many, only three colors, red, yellow and blue, are fine. Even black pencil will also be OK.

Before the patient starts, first explain that by naturally moving your eyes as you follow the line in the drawing exercise, your brain will manage to loosen tangled thought.

Form Drawing Technique
From Straight Lines to Wavy Lines

Place the paper sideways and start from the upper left (for left-handers start from the upper right).

Relax your shoulders.

Let's Start!

Imagining the huge sky and sea,

draw a straight line from left to right.

Draw another one between the distant sky and the sea.

Then draw another one.

The wind has started to blow.

Draw slightly wavy lines.

The wind has started to blow harder.

Draw naturally larger wavy lines.

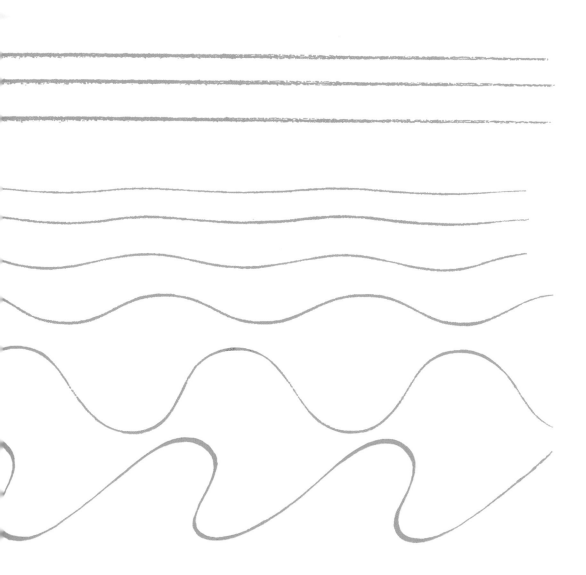

Prepare another piece of paper.
This time, draw large wavy lines first, and then go back to drawing straight lines.

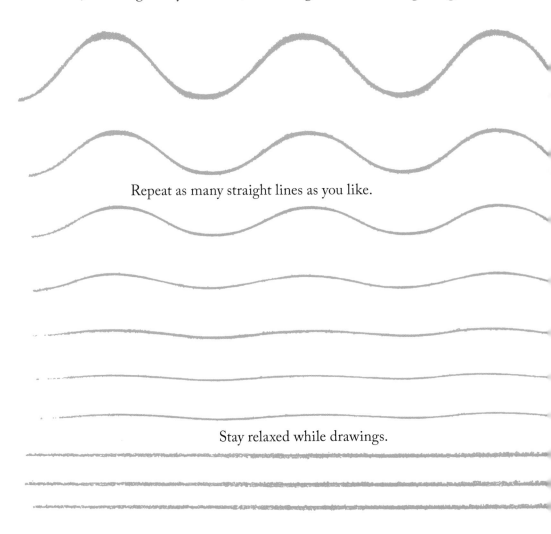

Repeat as many straight lines as you like.

Stay relaxed while drawings.

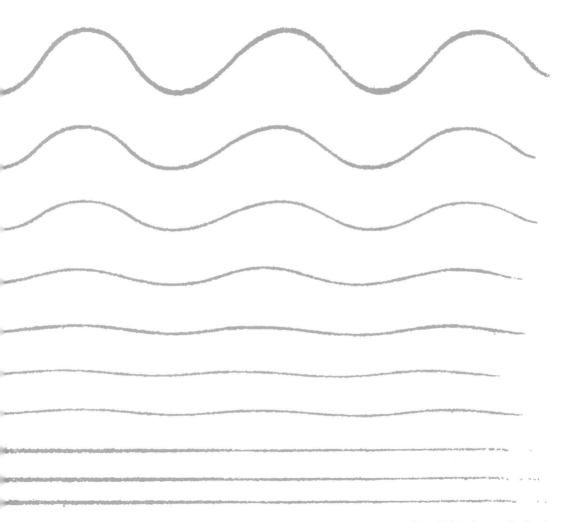

Source "A Line Drawing The Time"

Next Drawing Sideways Figure 8s.

Place the pencil in the middle of paper and draw a circle right or left, up or down, as you like. When you come back to the starting point, draw a circle to the other side and come back to the starting point.

You've made a sideways figure 8.

Use different colors and go over the same sideways figure 8.

Repeat as many times as you like.

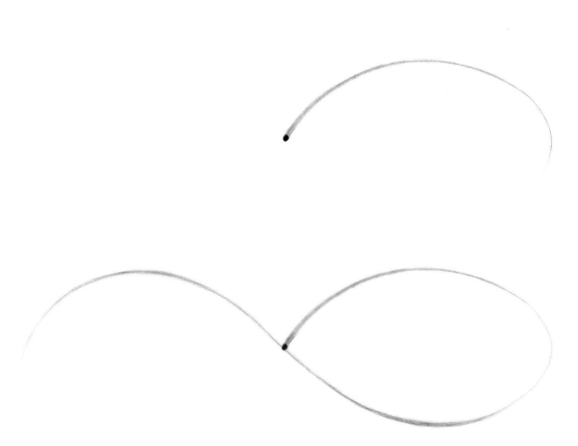

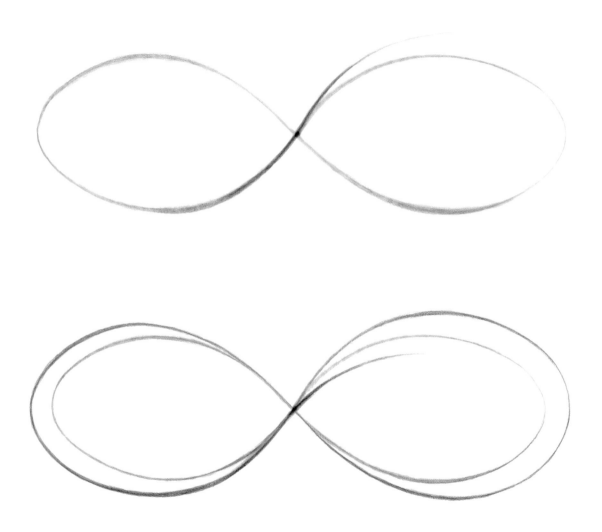

You can draw as if you were a driver on a racing circuit.

You can't crash.

Keep your eyes on the lines.

Draw 8s

Place the paper vertically.

Place the pencil at about the middle of the paper.

Draw a circle downwards, go back to the starting point, and then draw a circle up in the sky.

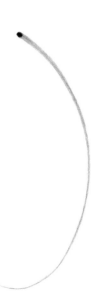

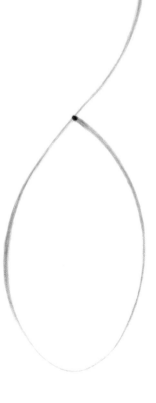

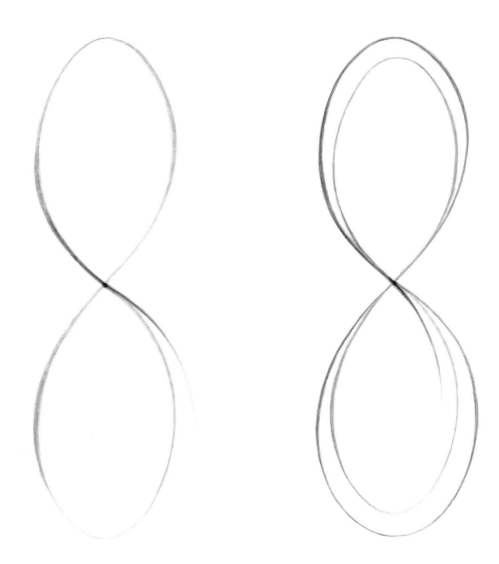

Repeat as many times as you wish while exhaling.

When you get used to it, combine the sideways 8 and the 8 together (it looks like a fat cross), and repeat them as many times as you wish.

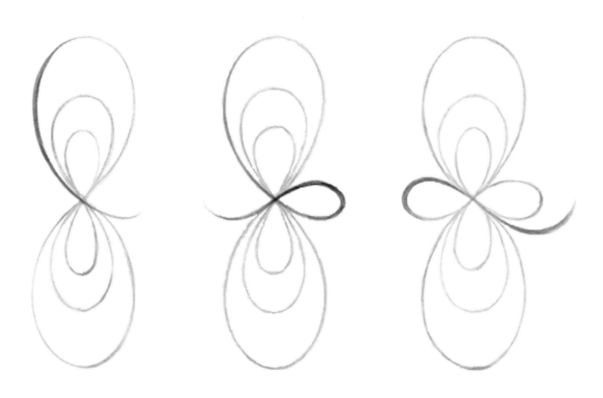

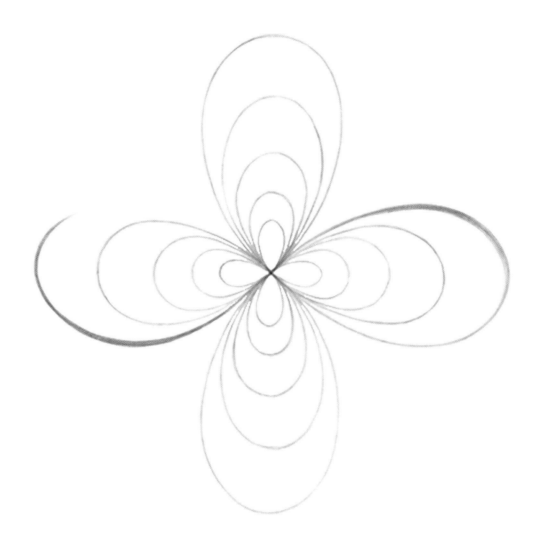

Children's Form Drawings

Straight Lines to Wavy Lines

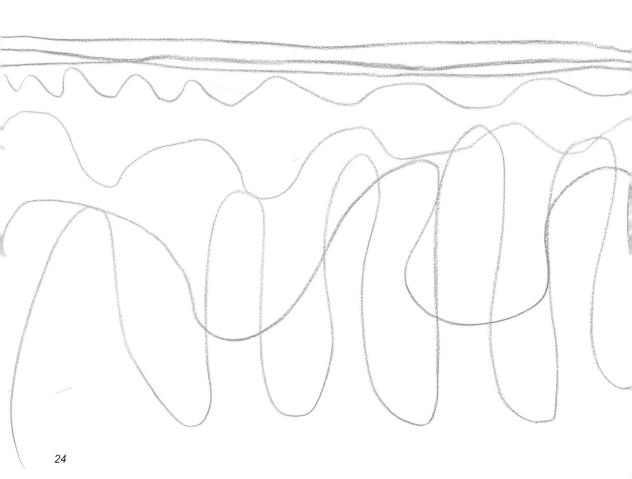

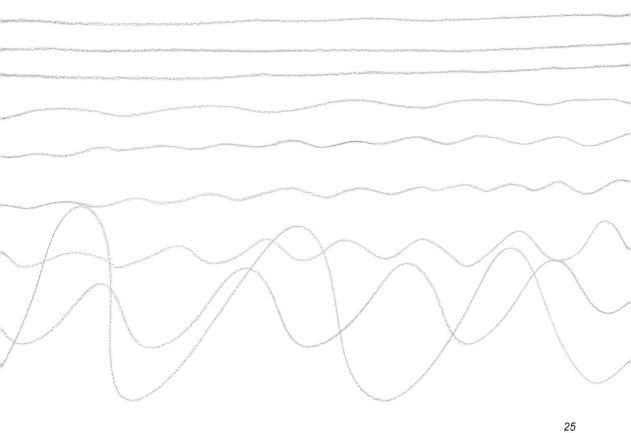

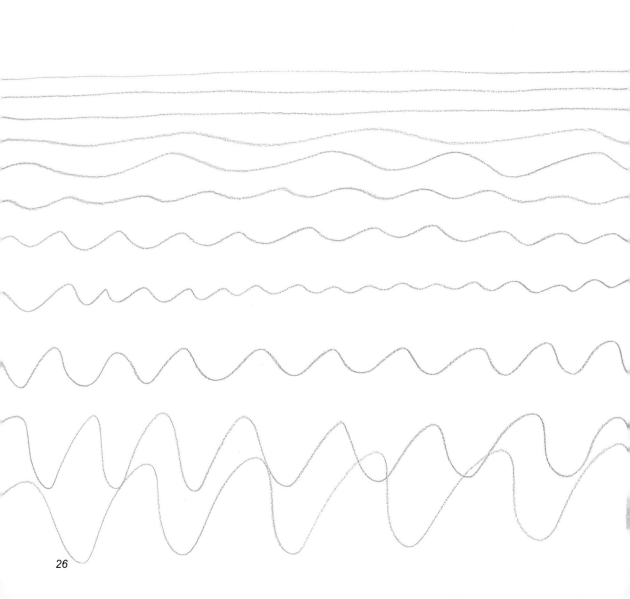

"When I started drawing wavy lines,

I felt as if I was floating in my mother's womb."

This was a comment by a seventeen-year-old girl.

Drawing 8s

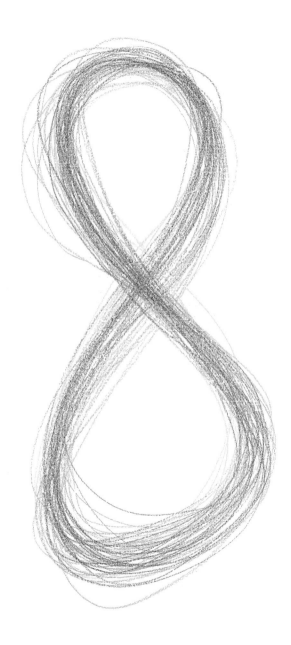

"When I drew fast, I did not think about
 anything."
"It was fun."
It was as if negative ideas had disappeared.

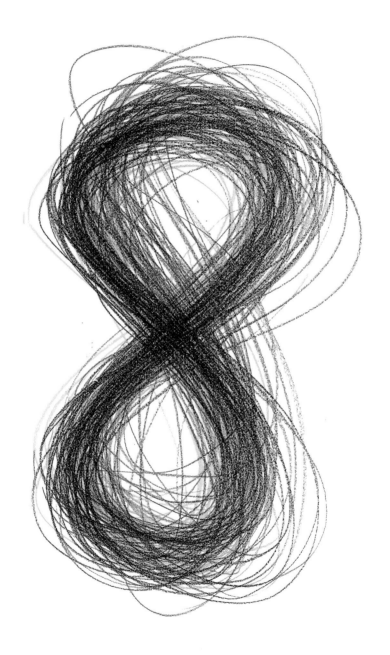

When you start drawing you should draw slowly, but to
 enhance your eye movement, draw rapidly.
Do not worry about messy lines.

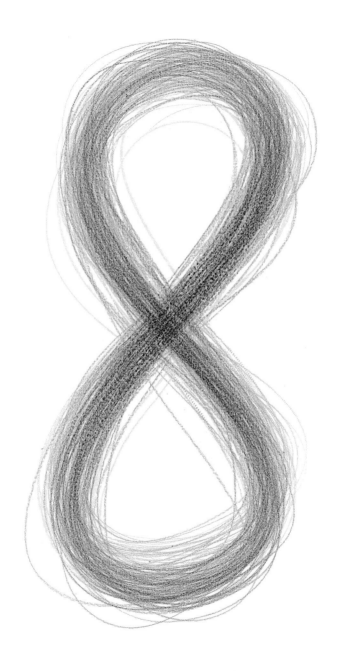

Sometimes you become sleepy suddenly.
In such a case, you say out loud,
"Five, four, three, two, one, wake up!"
This is a good sign; when you make yourself sleepy,
 it means you've concentrated enough so that you are
freed from negative thoughts.

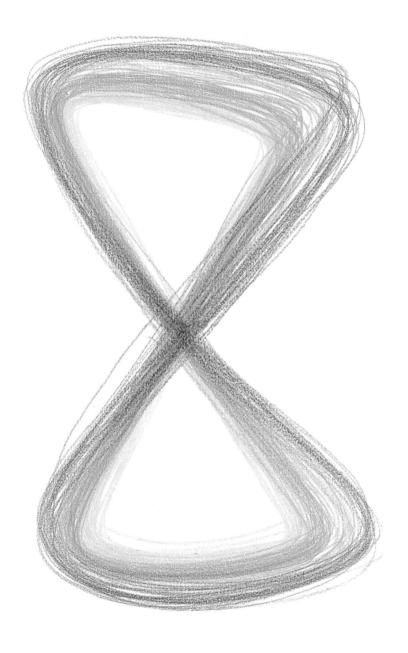

When you finish drawing, write down whatever you felt in the corner of paper.
This makes you realize what changes actually occurred.

Variety of Shapes

The figure 8 has a variety of shapes, and it's color and the pressure vary depending on the patient's mental status. Generally, at first, tension and inexperience results in weak color and weak pressure, but when trust in the examiner develops, the form becomes free and the color and pressure become stronger.

On recovery, the pressure and the colors become lighter and the number of times the figure is repeated tends to decrease. After drawing, patients can write their feelings in the corner of the paper. The patients' feelings are important because they try to think for themselves about their mental issues. Our work begins at this point.

For M-REMB, remind the patient that it is important that both eyes move smoothly and that the up/down and right/left balances are important. His eyes should follow the line drawings naturally.

Start counting the numbers together with the patient, go over 100, 500 and 1,000 times. The patients' obsessions, worry, and fear are freed, and their faces become bright. We found that by applying M-REMB, the effect of release was enhanced and the treatment duration was shortened.

The trauma is different for each individual, but for toddlers, enjoyment and concentration are important. We found it necessary to remind them what they are doing.

For adults and adolescents, in order to continue the treatments, we found it important to explain the importance of M-REMB to the patients.

Chapter II

Image Breathing

Image Breathing: Towards Deep Breathing

People have long known that deep breathing is soothing.

Sometimes you stop breathing when you're shocked. Sometimes you take shallow breaths due to anxiety. When patients who suffer from overwhelmingly strong images have negative thoughts while doing line drawings, their breathing becomes shallow.

For adults and toddlers, we applied a breathing technique that we developed called "Image Breathing" and we found that it improved the effect.

It is a combination of breathing in, holding and breathing out.

If the total duration was long, they suffered from the lack of mental and physical energy, so we found that a pattern of breathing in for five seconds, holding for five seconds, and breathing out for five seconds should be done more than 3 times.

Adding to these breathing techniques, we found imagining images turned out to be successful.

Have the patient place both hands on their navel, and depending on their age and the circumstances, have them imagine cool, clear air.

For example, say, "You are breathing in clear air beside a waterfall and negative ions are around you."

For toddlers, you might say, "You are drinking some nice, cool juice."

While they are breathing in for 5 seconds, you say, "Breathe in clean air that cleanses your entire body."

While they are holding for five seconds, you say, "Place the most important thing in your abdomen."

While they are breathing out for five seconds, you say "Breathe the scary, negative, and dirty things out through your mouth."

By so doing, you can encourage your patients to breathe deeply and long.

Image Breathing can be done standing, sitting or lying down.

Sometimes it is better to let the patient lie down.

When they say, "I fell asleep." it is the best thing that can happen.

Image Breathing Technique

Place both hands on your navel, and imagine placing something very important there — something that will save you from anything that scares you.

Now let's begin.

(1) Breath out by shrinking your abdomen.

(2) Relax your abdomen and let the air flow into your lungs.

(3) Hold your breath for three to five seconds (the longer, the better).

(4) Breathe out for about five seconds (the longer, the better). Cleanse your body of whatever scary, negative, or dirty things there might be. Then go back to (2) above.

Repeat this "Image Breathing" 3 times.

Focus on the important thing you placed on your navel. Your abdomen will become warn and you will become more and more relieved.

How was it? Did you get rid of a lot of anxiety? I imagine some of you have successfully released your anxiety.

In the following part, we will show the successful results of a number of cases. We dealt with such cases as PTSD (50 cases), obsessive-compulsive disorder (52 cases), others (20 cases). The age distribution is below ten years old (11 cases), above ten years (52 cases), and above twenty years (32 cases). We will show typical results.

Chapter III

Children Who Were Released from Trauma (PTSD)

Trauma Caused by Child Abuse

The Case of A

A was a 4-year-old girl. Her young single mother used to disappear often, during which time A was raised by her grandparents. She suffered from fake coughs. Her single mother got married. As a results she stayed with new parents. Her nursery school teacher realized then that she suffered from child abuse.

She said her father was scary — he bit and kicked her. Thus her grandparents started to look after her. Still her fake coughing continued. Pediatricians suggested these symptoms must be coming from some mental cause. Her grandmother brought her to our clinic.

They were apparently the results of abuse by her stepfather.

We started M-REMB on the first day.

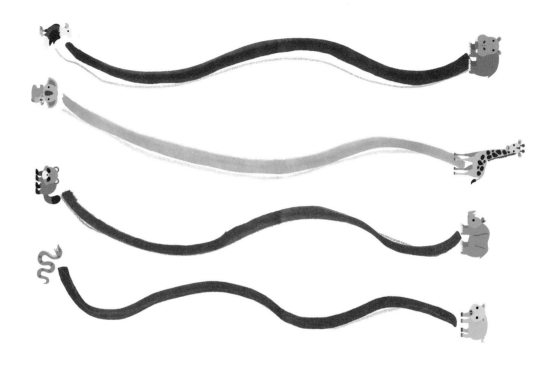

Since she is still a toddler, it was difficult using the same paper work.
When drawing a straight line from left to right, we pasted two seals
at both ends and let her connect them along with markers.

Next, we got her to connect panda to panda.

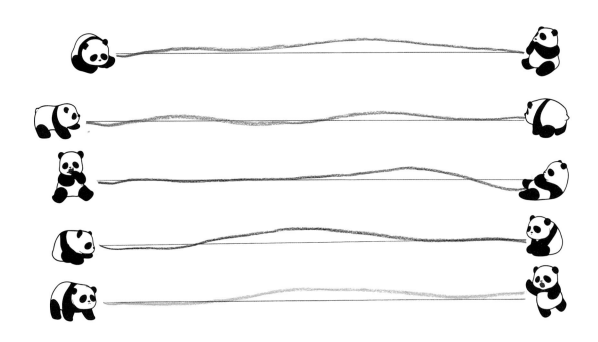

At last, she had done her straight lines and wavy lines by herself!

Next, she drew 8s.

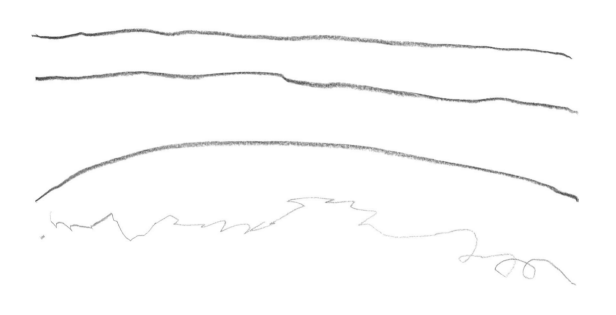

When drawing a sideways 8, it seemed difficult for her,
a toddler, to cross the line.

She drew two circles and gourd shapes, but when she
managed to draw the crossing, she seemed to have managed
to jump over a stream, and she seemed to be released.

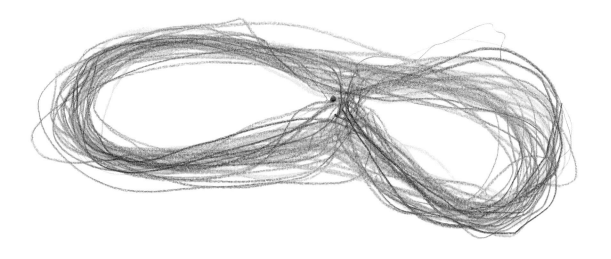

53

Next, she seemed to have not lost her way in drawing 8s, and eventually managed to cross the lines.

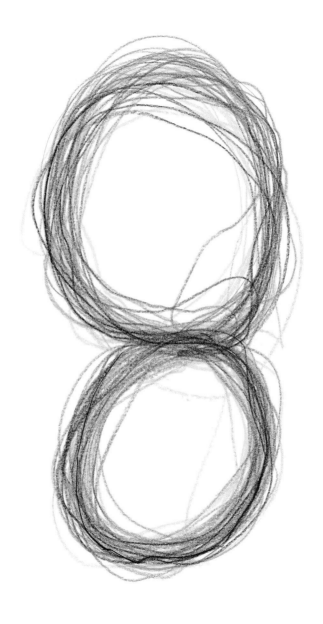

After starting Form Drawing, her fake coughs disappeared. We asked her grandparents to remove her from her mother's care, and we also asked the nursery school to cooperate.

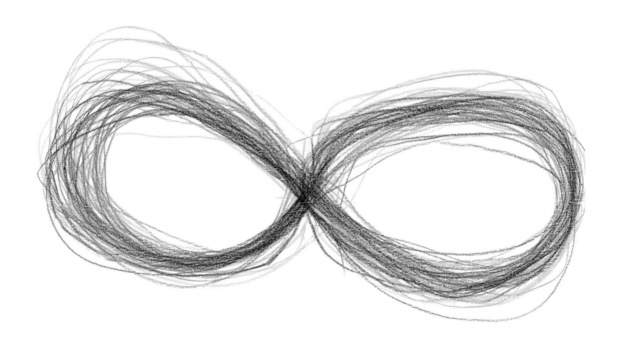

For the last visit to our clinic, she drew standing and sideways 8s well and seemed to enjoy it.
Her fake coughs disappeared completely.
At the first visit, she used to act like a baby, but after treatment, the need to suck at her mother's breast had completely disappeared.

Thus, she graduated from our clinic.

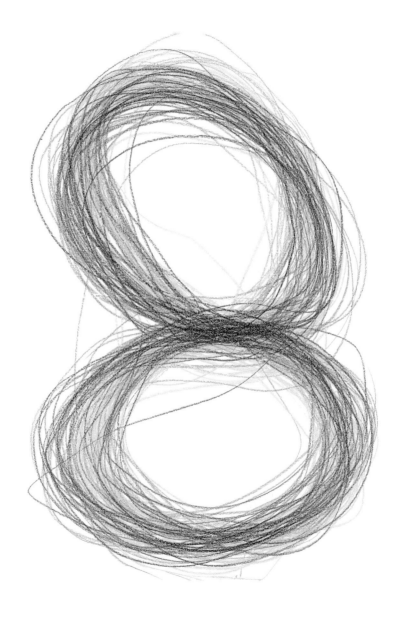

The disorder because of Domestic violence

The Case of B

From the beginning, the 6-year-old girl drew a figure 8 more than 1,000 times.

Her father yelled at her mother, and her mother used Girl B as a shield. The mother and the daughter escaped from the father, and apparently a divorce proceeding is ongoing.

When she started school, she was scared of the class teacher. She was scared to go to the washroom, but the teacher's reaction was harsh.

At the first visit to our clinic, she was scared of strange people in the clinic. And her grandparents and I had to escort her to the treatment room. Namely the object of her fear widened from her father to people and to school and to strangers. This is a typical case of PTSD caused by the father's yelling.

Line drawings started timidly at first, but she drew a sideways 8 301 times, and she drew 8s 1,085 times.

"Interesting" and "enjoyable," she uttered.

At this time, she must have been released from her fear. On the way home, she was not afraid of people any more, and went home without showing any fear to people.

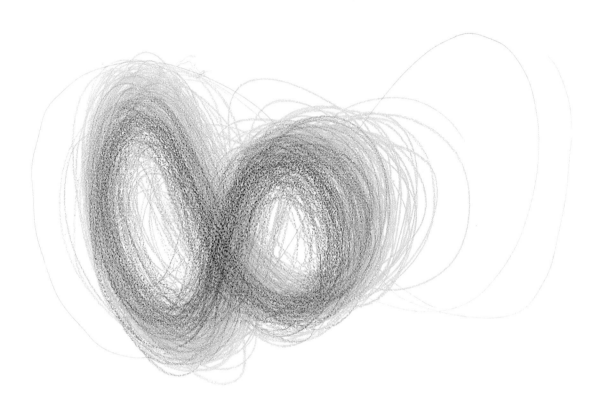

62

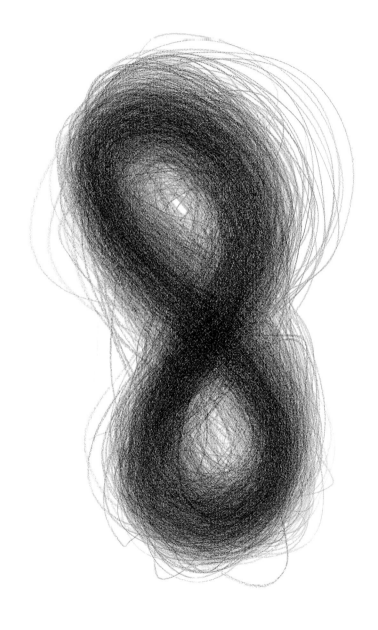

At the fourth session, she drew both 8s 400 times. She said she did not think anything.

After the session, she joined in an outdoor activity and went home smiling.

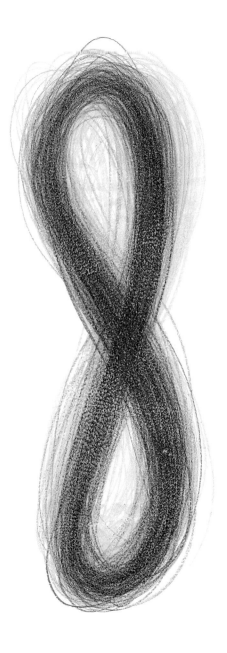

At the fifth session, she graduated from the clinic.

She drew both **8**s 400 times, and she drew a picture about the session.

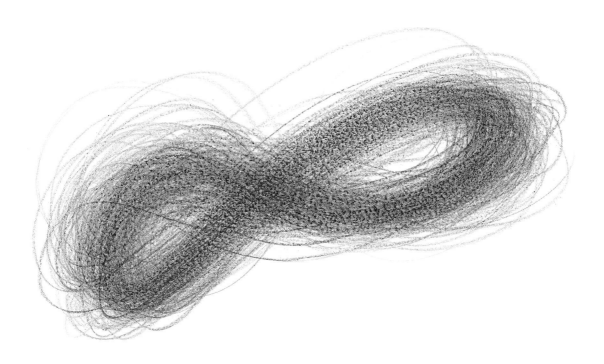

Drawing 8s 300 to 1,000 times seemed to make her free from fear.

Her mother divorced her father, and she lived safely. Girl B made friends, and she can now tolerate the scary teacher.
At the end of 3 months, she graduated from the clinic.

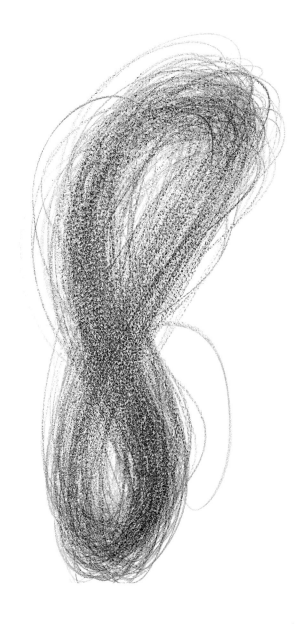

Trauma Caused by Natural Disasters

Victim of Flooding

The Case of C

When a huge flood struck, Boy C was 6 years old. When he and his mother went into the house from the parking lot, water was up to their navels. His father came to rescue them, but he did not succeed. They had to wait for 6 hours to be rescued. They were rescued by a boat and stayed in the evacuation center for 2 days.

After one year passed, at nights he started to cry. He could not go out. In the house he could not walk on the floor; he stood on the chair and could do nothing but yell. His grandmother came to help. But his mother and he both showed fear of water.

From the beginning, we tried M-REMB on both. At first, he did not look into the eyes of our staff members, and to questions and indications, he uttered quietly, "Yes." He stared at the paper on the desk. He chose blue. He drew straight lines and wavy lines. The shape of the wavy lines was drawn carefully. He must have been tense.

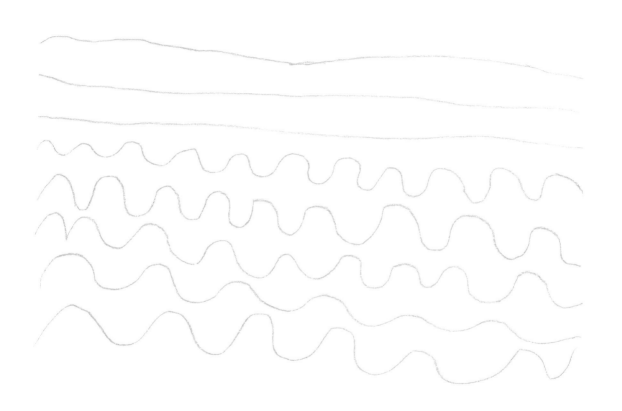

When he was drawing sideways figure 8s, he uttered "enjoyable" and "happy."
He drew 8s quickly, and he did it more than 200 times.

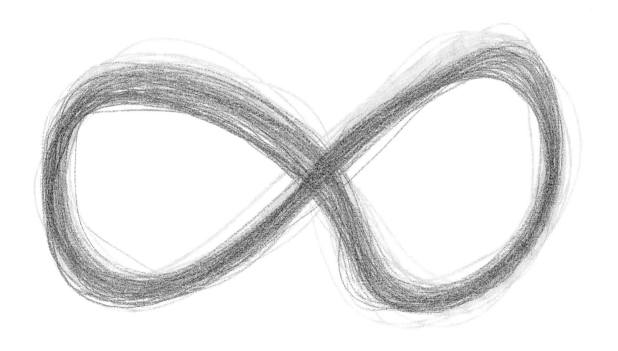

At the next visit, I was surprised to see his straight lines were stable and his wavy lines were written freely.

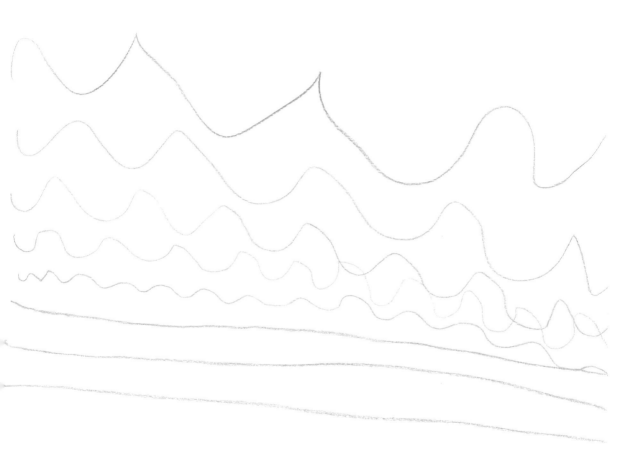

He drew 8s 100 to more than 200 times.
He uttered, "I did not think anything."
"I did enough."
And "I liked the color I used."

On the way home he said, "I am not afraid of rain
drops or the noise of the wind."

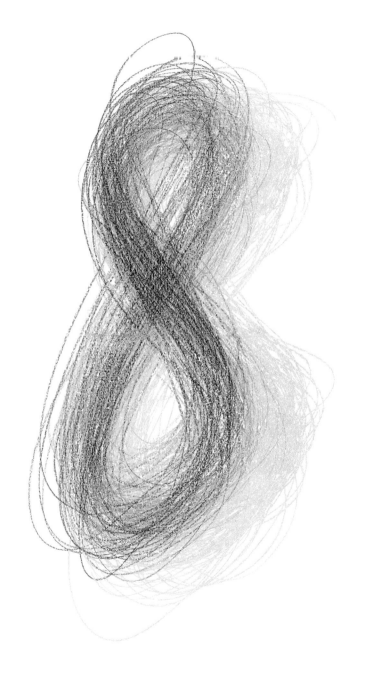

At the third visit, he changed so much that he talked about his school, about his friends, about his best subject.

Although he was still afraid of thunderstorms, he said his fear of floods had shrunk to about "this much," and he gestured with his hands about 10 cm apart.

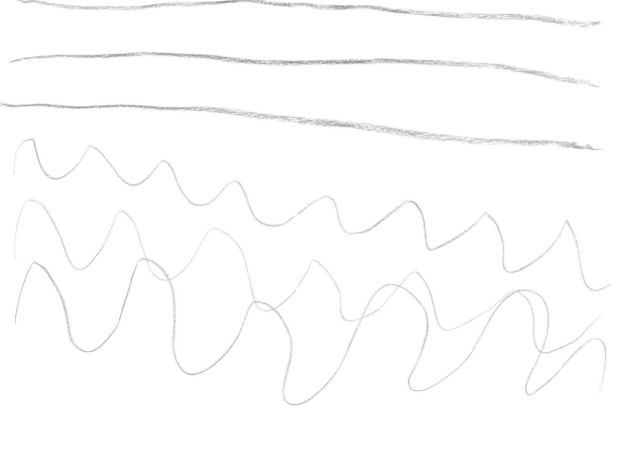

At the fourth visit, he drew forms freely, and said, "It was enjoyable."

He also said, "I could not swim in the sea, but I could swim in a pool."

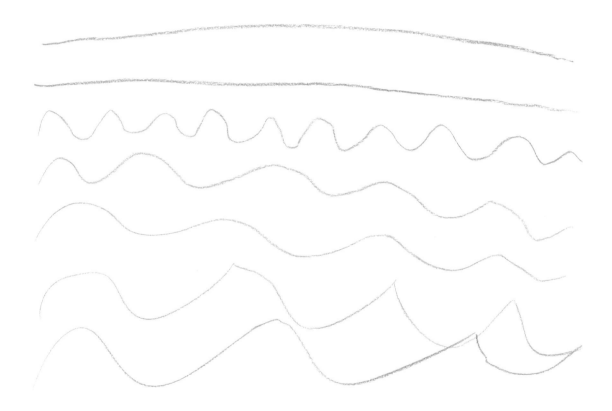

He was enthusiastic about Form Drawing from the beginning.
He was a case of quick recovery.

In his family life, his father helped him with Form Drawing, and he drew 8s every day.

Suffered from East JAPAN Disaster in IBARAKI

The Case of D

The 9-year-old girl came to the clinic. She was scared of the dark, was scared of confined spaces, had nightmares, and thus she wanted to die.

The cause of all these was the East Japan Disaster that had happened when she was 3 years old. After that, she refused to go to kindergarten, and she refused to go to school. The night before the first visit, she cried often, "I want to die."

I diagnosed her as having had PTSD for 7 years, and I started M-REMB.

At first, she drew a sideways figure 8 quietly.

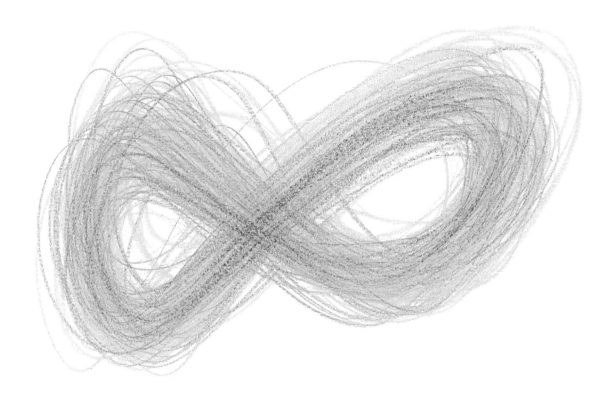

She kept drawing both 8s quickly.

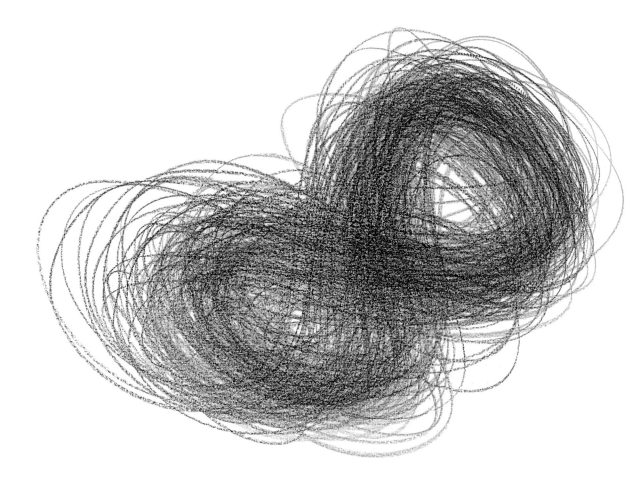

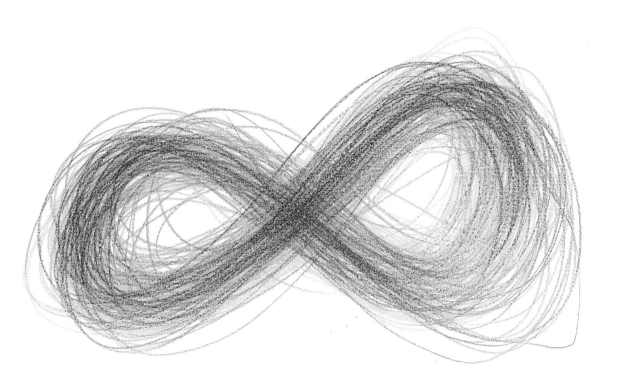

After 6 months, she started to talk about the fear of earthquakes.

At this time, she used bright colors.

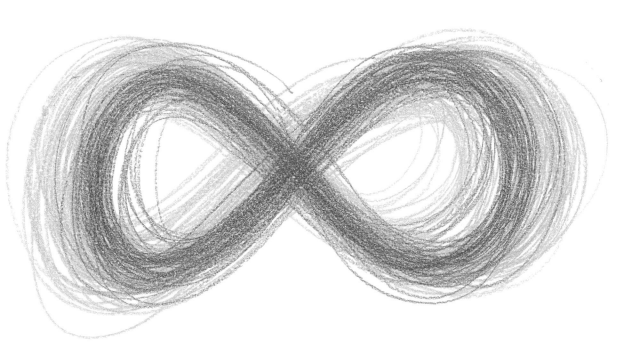

After nine months, she said, "I do not dream scary dreams any longer," and she joined in outdoor activities. Then after twelve months, she graduated from the clinic.

The reason why she did not show the quick recovery was that her mother was suffering from panic disorder. But weekly sessions for twelve months set her free from her fear. She drew 8s 14,400 times in all, in the twelve months.

Suffered from East JAPAN Disaster in FUKUSHIMA

The Case of E

The East Japan Disaster was also the cause of her PTSD. She was an eleven-year-old girl at the first visit.

At the age of five, she experienced the East Japan Disaster while living in Fukushima City. Food and drinking water were in short supply, meaning that long line-ups were necessary. Her mother was pregnant. She suffered from morning sickness and could not drink water. She almost miscarried. Thus, she had to rest.

Girl E did not talk among excited adults, could not go to the washroom, and could not leave her mother's side. She could not make friends for more than six months. At one time, they both stayed at her grandmother's house, and she changed kindergartens. But after three months, her younger sister was born with a deformity in her heart.

The baby had heart surgery and the girl had eye surgery at about the same time.

One year after the East Japan Disaster, her father was moved to the Okinawa area, and she started school there. Then, she received a precise examination which found that she had a Developmental Disorder (This is a name of special kind of Mental Retardation.) and has some difficulty living in a group setting.

She needed special help to live in a group, because it was difficult for her to communicate with people.

She withdrew and became attached to her mother. Medical clinics prescribed a medicine for Developmental disorder. Each time she moved, she changed hospitals.

At the first visit to our clinic, she was eleven years old. M-REMB was introduced. Since Girl E shows fear, we asked her mother to join her in the treatment room. Girl E sat on the floor, stuck to her mother's legs, brushed away the pencils, and stared at us with a hostile look.

Her mother held a pencil together with her, and they moved the pencil together. They continued together for a while, but eventually she took charge herself and kept counting sideways 8s more than 400 times. At this point something bothering her must have been released.

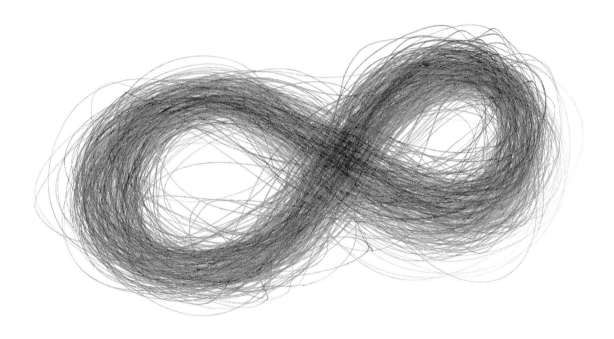

After a series of sessions were over, she went out by herself and found a swing and started to swing on it.

Her mother and I looked at each other with surprise.

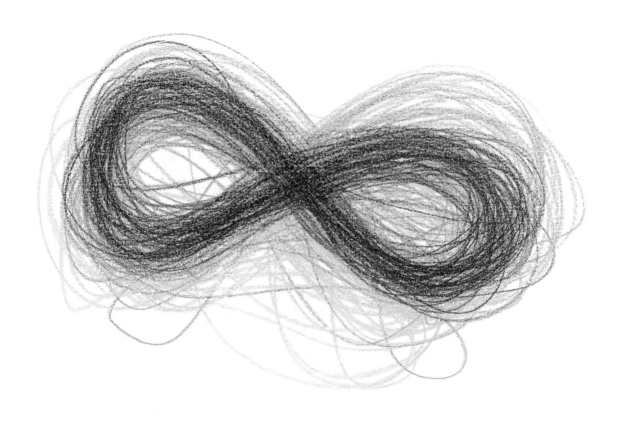

After repeated sessions, bright colors appeared.

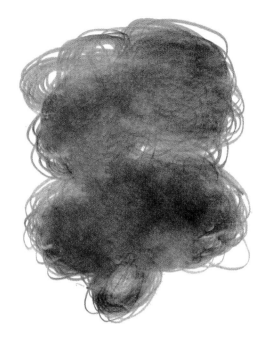

As homework, I told her to draw both 8s, and she did it a total of more than 2,000 times.

There must have been something bothering her, and she seemed to want to tell us.

At the fifth session, she drew both 8s a total of 800 times. After this, she had time to go out to play and ate pancakes and cookies.

She said, "I want to come back soon," and she reserved a session for the next week.

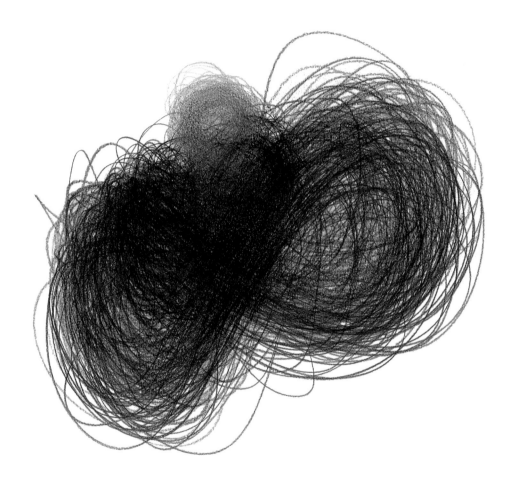

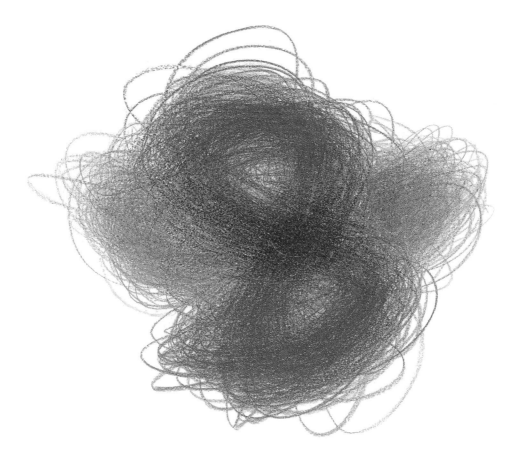

For seven years, she could not go to the washroom without her mother.
But at the sixth session, she was able to go to the washroom with a
staff member of the clinic. On that day she drew above.

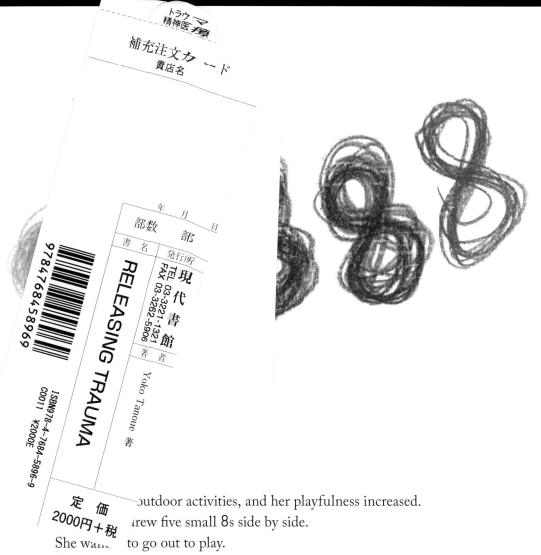

トラウマ
精神医房

補充注文カード
貴店名

年　月　日
部数　　部
書名　　発行所
現代書館
TEL 03-3221-1321
FAX 03-3262-5906
著者

RELEASING TRAUMA

Yoko Tanoue 著

9784768458969

ISBN978-4-7684-5896-9
C0011 ¥2000E

定価
2000円＋税

...outdoor activities, and her playfulness increased.

...rew five small 8s side by side.

She wan... to go out to play.

That seemed to be her announcement of graduation from Form Drawing.

The more exciting things she wanted to do were activities in nature.

When snow fell, she made a "Kamakura (an igloo)." She also went into the bushes and made a "secret base." She asked her mother, "I want you to help me, when I need it in school."

In March, for those who cannot attend the graduation ceremony at school, we plan an event at our clinic called "Celebration of Spring." At that event, she sang a song in front of people. Our staff was surprised, and we watched the video of her singing again and again.

Before the East Japan Disaster, she had enjoyed kindergarten. But repeated traumatic experiences, such as destruction by a once-in-a-thousand-years earthquake, radioactive pollution from the destruction of a nuclear power plant by the huge tsunami, changing schools after fleeing from the pollution, her younger sister's surgery and her own surgery, apparently overwhelmed her. Visits to hospitals over five years did not help her. After six years, she was released from the trauma. After each M-REMB sessions, outdoor experiences also helped her.

Chapter IV

Other Cases

Those children who were brought to the clinic tended to have fear, negative thoughts and anger towards adults and society. They cannot swallow even medicine. In order to remove anxiety or fear, we used M-REMB, and we found that other psychological treatments were not useful for obsessive-compulsive disorders or stuttering, but we show by using M-REMB, we succeeded.

Obsessive-Compulsive Disorder

The Case of F

The eight-year-old boy, who suffered from this symptom, tended to think something one should not think, for example, this Boy F said, "Mother you should die." Having heard this, his mother was shocked and brought the boy to our clinic.

He does not know the seriousness of "death." That's why children utter such words very often. So we started M-REMB.

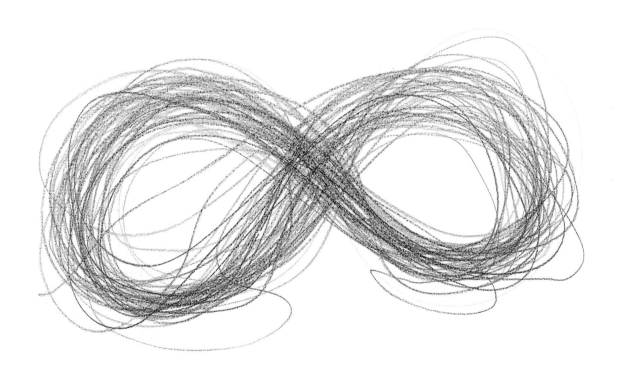

At the first session he drew both 8s.

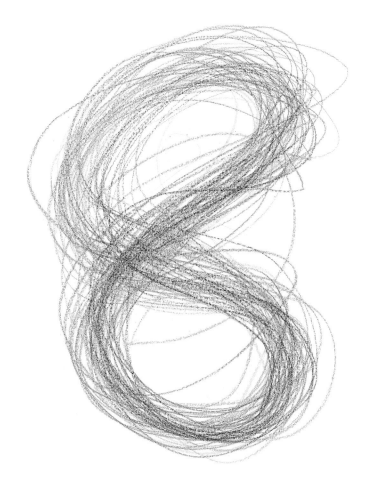

When he finished, he told something that had been bothering
him since he was six years old, even his mother did not know.

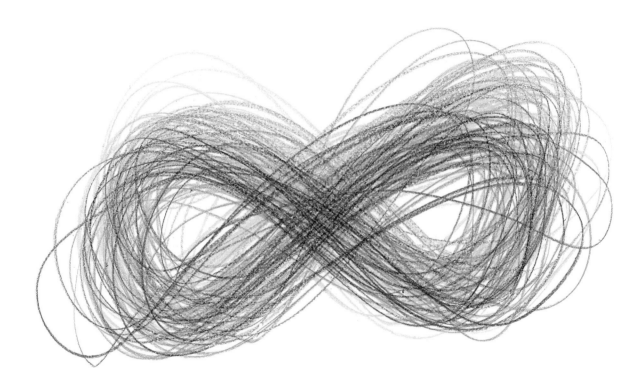

At the second session, he drew **8**s with some bright colors, impetuously.

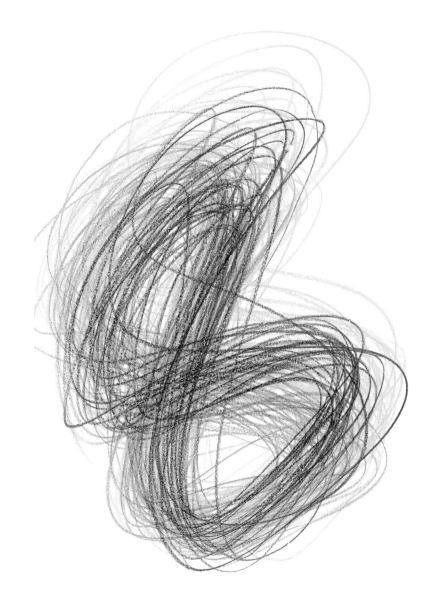

After 2 months, he used more bright colors, and drew 250 times.

While he drew 8s 250 times, his"death"must have been released.

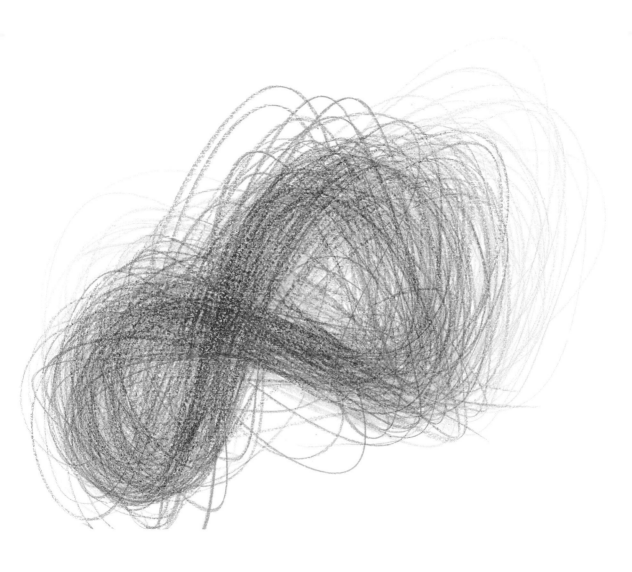

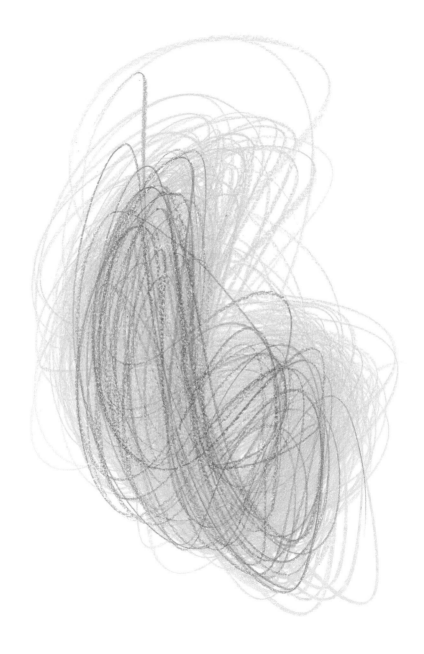

At the next visit, he said, "I did not think of death."
Of course, this was due in part to improvements in his environment because I had asked his teacher and parents not to interfere too much — not to scold him or criticize him too much — and to keep him relaxed.

After 2 more sessions, he graduated from our clinic.

Case of Stuttering

The Case of G

The ten-year-old boy came to the clinic with his father and grandmother. His stuttering was so bad that I could not understand what he said. His father had to translate what his son said for me.

When he read sentences, he skipped some sounds, words and sentences, here and there. Communication must have been difficult for him, and he must have had trouble making and keeping friends. M-REMB must work, I thought.

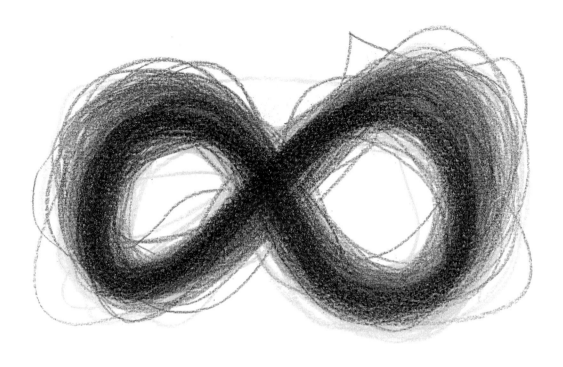

He drew sideways 8s 505 times and 8s 415 times. After Form Drawing, he had outdoor experiences and he moved with his father, during which time he did not suffer from stuttering.

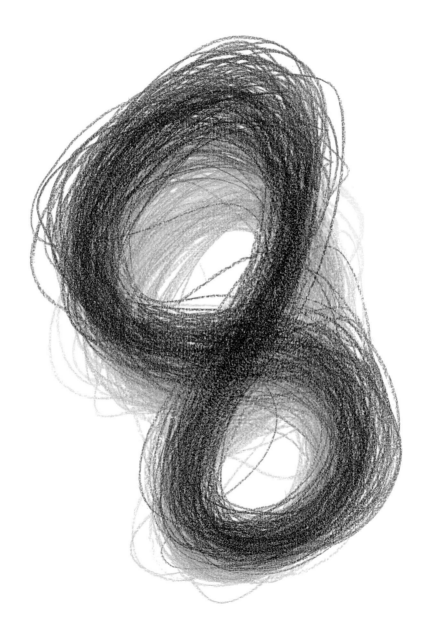

At the next session, he drew 8s 582 times. After the session he enjoyed outdoor activities, with barefoot.

"Wow! What a great feeling! This is my first time to play barefoot." This time his stuttering disappeared.

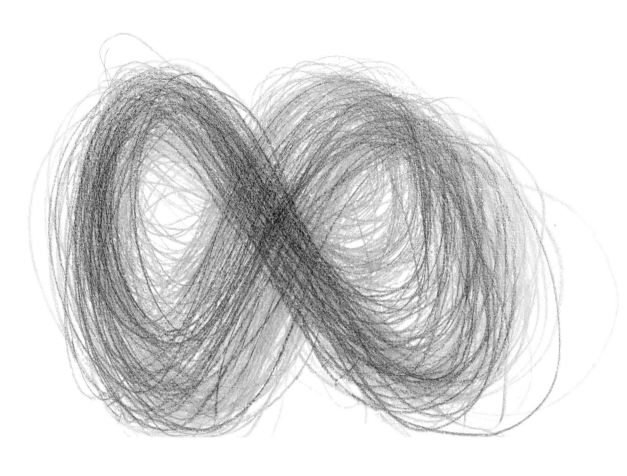

At home, he drew sideways 8s 904 times, and moreover, he used six colors.

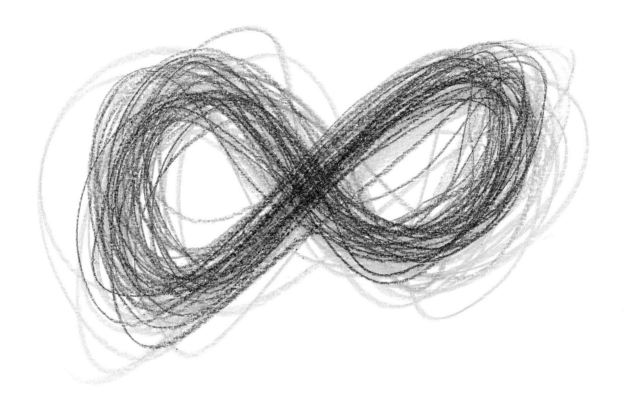

He eagerly came to the clinic, and he started to talk a lot.

Since he was an infant, he had been depressed because of his stuttering. He talked about friends with joy.

But now he talked about his mother, he said, "She calls me stupid G." It seemed his mother had an influence on his stuttering. It looked as if he was about to graduate, but then he had a fight with his mother, and he started stuttering again. But this time, he managed to conquer his stuttering with M-REMB. He realized that his problem was based on the relationship with his mother. After his fifth visit, he graduated from our clinic with the power of M-REMB.

For children, we found M-REMB was effective. In the next chapter, I will explain the jargon used by mental health professionals.

Chapter V

Explanation of Jargon and the Discovery of M-REMB

Post-Traumatic Stress Disorder (PTSD)

I will explain "PTSD" here. One branch of the United Nations, WHO, recognized the chronic illness caused by the outer reasons, Post Traumatic Stress Disorder (PTSD), in 1992. Such traumata caused non-reaction, or conversely cause violent reactions. Such reactions can be cured within a few days, but the patient does not remember what occurred during that period. After several weeks or months, the symptoms appear which are called PTSD. Typically, people with PTSD are tense, are surprised at minute sounds, cannot sleep, are excessively alert, have anxiety, and suffer from depression. Children with PTSD tend to cling to their mother's skirt, and they cannot sleep unless they sleep with their parents. They carry anxiety and depression, have no enthusiasm, and they do not laugh or cry.

They avoid the scene that reminds them of a traumatic event. For example, after the traffic accident, they are afraid of cars, and they do not want to ride in a car. Even though they avoid such situations, these traffic accidents come back as a flash back, and come back in their dreams.

While there are sometimes clear causes of PTSD, there are cases in which people suffer from PTSD without noticing the cause. Between husband and wife, children and parents, among friends, and between lovers, the damaged person tends to suffer from PTSD without noticing. Sometimes it causes death, or the person suffers from PTSD for years. Repeated attacks could cause peaceful minds to be lost and ending up with depression. Or it causes a negative spiral, which is slowly developing PTSD. Thus PTSD requires psychological treatment.

Modern Psychological Treatment

    Psychological treatment is said to have started by Sigmond Freud (1856-1939). Trauma means "injury" in the ancient Greek. And Freud used it as psychological connotation. Psychoanalysis was popular in the States and Europe, but it costs a lot and is also time consuming. Thus, varies type of behavior therapies were developed. Next, I will explain EMDR, which was what caused me to write this book.

EMDR (Eye Movement Desensitization and Reprocessing.)

In 1989, Francine Shapiro discovered EMDR. She accidentally moved her eyeballs quickly, and she realized that what she was suffering from had disappeared. After the Vietnam War, a large number of former soldiers suffered from various forms of PTSD, and there was an urgent need for a cure.

She published a book entitled "Eye movement desensitization and reprocessing : Basic principles, protocols and procedures, " in 1995. In short, EMDR is to remind the patient the reason for his trauma. The method of eyeball movement is for the examiner to hold two fingers in front of the patient, and move them left to right, up and down, making sure that the patient follows his fingers while increasing their speed gradually.

It is important that both eyeballs follow the examiner's fingers. Each time, check whether the degree of anxiety is reduced or not. A few times was enough for some cases, but other cases required a few years.

The human brain is awake when one is asleep. While one is asleep, eyeballs are moving rapidly. We call this type of sleep REM (Rapid Eye Movement) sleep. Though it is not yet fully understood, it has said that one's brain remains busy, managing information. During EMDR we make patient's brain mimic this state and untie the tangled thoughts.

This method was groundbreaking, but it was not necessarily perfect. Depending on the patient, it had some flaws. Thus we established a Psychological Treatment.

From EMDR to M-REMB

EMDR was developed, ending up with M-REMB. Counselor Midori Maki attend the seminar of joined Trauma Therapy in both 2007 and 2009 held in Germany. She was licensed. We started using EMDR in October 2009 at our clinic.

I felt it has a limit. It is because EMDR reminds the patient of the reasons for PTSD, which can be painful. I decided that removing the part of reminding the reasons for trauma can also be effective. Another problem is that for toddlers and for persons of advanced years, who have psychiatric disease, they tend to feel uncomfortable doing quick eye movements, and its usage has its own limitation.

While I was searching for answers, I found that Steiner education's Form Drawing was a great hint. Namely, we started Form Drawing. When we're drawing lines, our eyeballs move smoothly without much efforts. Eyeballs movements are not forced, and we don't notice we're doing it. By drawing lines enthusiastically, the patient releases their stress.

Next, I realized breathing technique is important. Most of our patients tend to take shallow breaths. We realized that the patients can breathe without much efforts, and we arrive at Image Breathing.

Keep both hands on the navel. Breath in clean air. Under both hands place the most important things and hold your breath. Slowly breathe out fear and negative thoughts in order to cleanse them from your body.

Remembering important things within the patient works well in relieving fear. Their important things could be, "God," "the sun," "parents," "favorite books," "stuffed dolls," etc. As they place these images, they can start deep breathing. As mentioned above, in EMDR, they have to tell the degree of fear, but the patients refused violently at first. Instead, we thus deleted the part in which we remind them the causes of trauma. Thus we succeeded in relieving them and let them start talking about their problems. With this Image Breathing, confusion within themselves eventually sorted out, and they started to talk about their fears. They can talk about the trauma when the trauma was washed away. We only listen and chime in once in a while.

After this happens, if they wish they can do the outdoor activities. Then the session is over, and they reserve the next session. This method is now called **M**ental **R**elease by **E**ye **M**ovement and **B**reathing (**M-REMB**), which was named by Emeritus Professor of Kyushu University Taichi Maki.

Steiner Education and Form Drawing

Form drawing was originated by Rudolf Steiner (1869-1925). Steiner took education as art and applied education as well as art to develop infant education. He succeeded in medical treatment and agriculture. He studied deeply Goethe's Color Study and thus that became the starting point. Steiner School was established in Waldorf 1919. Depending on children's stages of development, primary, middle, and high schools consistent education. Over thirty years ago in our clinic, we introduced classes of water colors and pastel using three primary colors, in which Form Drawing was introduced.

The classes that concentrate on line drawings were popular. Steiner applied Form Drawing to first grade pupils. He said, "Children feel various forms in their minds, and by actually drawing on a piece of paper, they can experience it internally. Thus, their emotions move, and their thoughts develop. Their minds become one through Form Drawing." (Helmut Eller, translated by Masayo Toriyama.)

These line drawings become simpler, Masako Kosuge wrote a book, "A Line Drawing The Time" that was published in 2003. This book emphasizes playfulness, and has some connections towards ancient drawings. We applied these to M-REMB.

Postscript

In Ushiku City, IBARAKI Prefecture, I have operated a clinic for thirty years. I announced M-REMB for the first time in 2014 at the annual meeting held in IBABAKI Prefecture. M-REMB gathered attention. In 2016, Seiichi Harada edited "Out Patient Psychological Series," and "On EMDR's Simple Development by Joining Image Respiration Method." was published. After that we announced and published about M-REMB a few times. The readers who read all these papers requested a simpler and easy-to-read book. Thus, I started to write this book. (Those are all Japanese.)

Natural disaster can occurs at any moment. While the government can look after us, we have to look after ourselves. Are you preparing foods for refuge and an escape route? How about the psychological part? But the psychological care is way behind. Those who have read this book, when you meet calamity, fight back by using M-REMB.

Please spread the word about M-REMB to children and people you know. As introduced in this book, drawing lines with many colors 200 times or 500 times will help you clear your mind. If you don't have any pencils, you can draw on the ground with nearby sticks. If you are in bed, you can draw in the air with your fingers. In the last two situations, I recommend draw sideways figure 8s only. Men can live with light and hope. The examples shown in this book were approved by the family members. Sideways 8s are full of infinite possibilities.

The drawings by children were all collected by Midori Maki with a lot of patience. Before treatments, the patients who were frozen by fear came out within an hour smiling, such is the magical staff. I pay tribute to them for their love and patience.

Ms. Masako Kosuge worked as a daycare teacher and helped us regarding the color play. She also wrote the explanation about the line drawings. I pay tribute to these two. For the long-awaited publication of this book, I thank Mr. Yasuhiro Kikuchi, Ms. Akiko Yamada, and Ms. Yuriko Amemiya.

Yoko Tanoue, M.D., Ph.D.

References

▶『EMDR──外傷記憶を処理する心理療法(Eye Movement Desensitization and Reprocessing)』
　Francine Shapiro 著、市井雅哉 監訳(二瓶社、2004年)　978-4861080081

▶『外来精神科診療シリーズ　パートⅡ　メンタルクリニックでの主要な精神疾患への対応(2)』
　森山成棯、原田誠一 編集(中山書店、2016年)　978-4521740041

▶『時を描く線　A Line Drawing The Time』小菅昌子 著(アトリエルピナス、2003年)

▶『フォルメン線描──こどもに対してEMDR施行時眼球運動の効果を上げる手法』
　田中麗香、真木みどり、田上洋子 共著(秋田精巧堂、2018年)

▶『人間を育てる』ヘルムート・エラー 著、鳥山雅代 訳(トランスビュー、2003年)　978-4901510110

▶『リトルブッダ』葉祥明 作・絵(佼成出版社、1996年)　978-4333017959

▶『ミュンヘンの小学生──娘が学んだシュタイナー学校』
　子安美知子 著(中公新書、1965年)　978-4121004161

▶『色彩論』ヨハン・ヴォルフガング・フォン・ゲーテ 著、木村直司 訳
　(ちくま学芸文庫、2001年)　978-4480086198

▶『エンデと語る──作品・半生・世界観』子安美知子 著(朝日選書、1986年)　978-4022594068

▶『モモ』ミヒャエル・エンデ 作、大島かおり 訳(岩波少年文庫、2005年)　978-4001141276

Author: Yoko Tanoue, M.D. , Ph.D.

Born in 1938. Graduated from Tokyo Medical Dental University in 1966. She worked as a child psychiatrist in hospitals,1990-2019 she has been taking care of children with psychiatric trouble in her office KODOMO NO SONO (which means play ground for children). She had a few articles about autistic children written in English. (Original English paper)

Translated into English by Yoshikata Koga, Ph.D.

Born in 1936. Graduated from Tokyo University in 1962. He studied 2more year after graduation. Responsible for Suiteki Juku (Water Drop Institute) and the Department of Chemistry, The University of British Columbia. His representative writing is [SOLUTION THERMODYNAMICS AND ITS APPLICATION TO AQUEOUS SOLUTIONS] He is a researcher of biophysical chemistry, and he translated this book for his grandchildren.

RELEASING TRAUMA

From EMDR to M-REMB

July 20, 2021　第 1 版第 1 刷発行

Author : Yoko Tanoue
Translator : Yoshikata Koga
Proofreader : Kathryn A. Craft
Publishing office : GENDAI SHOKAN PUBLISHING CO.,LTD.
　　　　　　　　3-2-5 Iidabashi, Chiyoda-ku, Tokyo 102-0072 Japan
　　　　　　　　Tel: +81-(0)3-3221-1321／Fax: +81-(0)3-3262-5906
Book design : Katsue Okutomi
Printed by : Hirakawa Kogyosha Co., Ltd.／Toko Insatsujo
Binder : Shinjudo Co., Ltd.
Collaborators : Midori Maki, Masako Kosuge (Atelier Lupinus) Tetsuya Oda

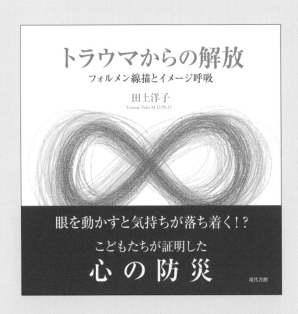